Table of Contents

Introduction

Ketogenic or keto diet is an interesting way to get rid of subcutaneous fat. On the one hand, you can eat almost no carbohydrates, but on the other, you can consume more fats, compared to what you are used to. With keto diet our body learns how to extract energy without using carbohydrates. When our body does not get carbohydrates (a way to get fast energy) at all, then ketones (ketone bodies) start to be produced from the fats to provide energy for the brain and nervous system. The process itself, when ketones are produced in our body, is called ketosis. It is the ketone bodies our brain starts to use as a source of energy instead of glucose.

This all might sound great, but the diets most of us are used to include a very high percentage of carbohydrates. This is partially due to the fact that many prefer to eat outside of home or consume other convenience foods. However, if you decided to follow keto diet to lose weight or for other health reasons, then you need to closely watch what you eat, including the number of calories received from carbohydrates, fats and proteins. To make your transition to keto diet easier and free you from counting calories, we created a 30-day keto meal plan for you.

In this 30-day keto meal plan, you will find that your breakfast, lunch, dinner and snacks and desserts are all planned out for you. We have included the amount of fat, net carbohydrates (carbohydrates minus fiber), and protein in each dish, so you can easily adjust your menu, if desired. Moreover, you can easily prepare every meal listed in the menu with the help of the simple to follow recipes included here. Keeping in mind that not everyone can cook every day, we also included meals that you can prepare ahead and freeze to enjoy later. Starting a keto diet just got much easier!

What is Keto Diet and How Does It Work

Keto diet is a diet with a limited intake of carbohydrates and a high content of fats and proteins. The main principle of this diet is more fat, less carbohydrates. This is one of the few known in our time diets, which allows you to get rid of fat while maintaining muscle mass. To visualize the mechanism of the keto diet, let us recall how the human metabolism is arranged. Carbohydrates are the main and most accessible source of energy. In conditions of limited intake of carbohydrates, the body is no longer able to receive energy by splitting carbs to glucose and is forced to use alternative sources of energy, i.e. fats, which are processed in the liver with formation of ketone bodies - this condition is called ketosis.

For most people, the very idea of eating fat to reduce weight seems paradoxical. However, the main goal of the keto diet is to make the body quickly change from glycolysis to lipolysis. Glycolysis is the process of splitting carbohydrates, and lipolysis - fat. Typically, carbohydrates are used, but with their lack, our body finds a solution and resorts to fats, which become the main source of energy. The latter is only triggered in the event of a complete depletion of glycogen in the liver and muscle tissue, usually in a few days. In the process of lipolysis, fats are split into free fatty acids and glycerin, which are subsequently transformed into ketone bodies. The process of formation of ketone bodies is called ketosis, hence the name of the diet itself.

In contrast with the usual low-carbohydrate diet, keto diet is longer and more systemic. In low-carbohydrate diets, carbohydrates can be consumed and usually this figure is more than 2 ounces, which is unacceptable for keto diet. With so many carbohydrates, the body cannot switch to continuous functioning on fats because processes related to ketosis do no occur. With keto diet, the body receives an insignificant amount of carbohydrates or they are completely absent from the diet, and it just has to function on fats. When you consume a lot of carbohydrates, only a certain part of them is absorbed in the intestines, and then it is split into simple sugars. After absorption, simple sugars increase the level of glucose in the blood, which provokes the secretion of insulin.

Insulin is able to enhance the synthesis of not only proteins, but also fats, so it is directly related to the accumulation of fat. At a time when insulin is high, it is able to prevent fat burning and storage of surplus nutrients in the fat cells. After a while, it can provoke a deficiency of glucose in the body, which will lead to a starvation. As a result of these processes, the brain sends signals and the person tries to fill the body with food as soon as possible. This is a constant cycle, which entails the processes of accumulation of fat. When you consume a low amount of carbohydrates, the blood glucose level rises gradually and often stabilizes, so there are no large increases of insulin. This approach, allows you to increase the breakdown of fat from fat stores, which leads to fat burning.

Keto diet can last from 2 to 3 weeks depending on the goals. It is possible to lose weight up to 22 pounds in just a month and you do not have to torment yourself with hunger. In the first week the body processes the reserves and adjusts to a new diet, and only starting from the second week it begins the process of ketosis, so if you plan to slightly reduce the weight and spend only a few days on it, keto diet is not for you. In this case, it is better to consider a simpler and more common low-carbohydrate diet. It is very important to correctly stop the keto diet and return to normal nutrition, gradually adding no more than 1 ounce of carbohydrates per day. Preparation of the body for ketosis takes place in 4 stages:

- **Total consumption of glucose.** The first 12 hours after the last meal the body spends glucose, derived from carbohydrates;
- **Total consumption of glycogen.** After 12 hours the body processes all the glucose and begins to draw supplies of glycogen from the liver and muscles. This phase lasts approximately 1-2 days;
- **Consumption of fats and protein.** This is the most difficult period, as having exhausted all the sources of carbohydrates, the body begins to process not only fatty acids, but also tries to get the necessary amount of glucose from protein. In this phase, the body tries to use protein, including muscle protein, as the main source of energy;
- **Ketosis, fat consumption.** This stage occurs, approximately, on the 7th day of the diet. The body adapts to the lack of carbohydrates and ketosis begins. The breakdown of protein in the body and food slows down and the main source of energy finally becomes fat.

For the proper functioning of the human body, three essential nutrients are vital: proteins, fats and carbohydrates. They are contained in ordinary food and each fulfills their functions:

- Fats are in a way a barrier between internal organs and are also accumulated for the "hard times";
- Proteins are the main building material for muscles, joints and the whole body. Without them, you can never build muscles and build a beautiful sculptured body. These organic substances are vital for professional athletes and all people, who lead an active lifestyle;
- Carbohydrates are the main source of energy. They give us cheerfulness and vitality.

Providing your body with moderate, proportionate amounts protein, fats and carbohydrates is equally valuable and necessary. That's why people, who are actively involved in sports and control their food intake, never have problems with being overweight. But if a person leads a sedentary lifestyle, regularly overeats or eats chaotically, often consumes fast foods, confectioneries and other sweets, it leads to excess fats and carbohydrates in the body, which are gradually transformed into fat storages under our skin or elsewhere.

Keto diet will help to lose weight and "cleanse" the body of excess fat. It will appeal to people, who find it difficult to limit themselves in food consumption and count calories. Before you go on this diet is important to consult a dietician and undergo a comprehensive examination of the body. Keto diet can give a tangible positive result, but only if the person is healthy. Keto diet is strictly prohibited for diabetics, pregnant women, people with thyroid gland issues, as well as for those, with kidney, liver and gastrointestinal tract problems.

Types of Keto Diet

The Standard Ketogenic Diet (SKD)is also referred to as "strict" keto diet and is the simplest and most recognized variety. It is just a very low carbohydrate, high fat and moderate protein diet. There are no carbohydrate loads(days with increased carbohydrates), the ratio of proteins, fats, and carbohydrates is constant (a lot of proteins and fats, few carbohydrates). It is suitable, if you can train well on low-carbohydrate diet or the trainings themselves are not very intense.

Targeted Ketogenic Diet (TKD) - carbohydrate loads are done in the periods before and after training. The goal of carbohydrate loading in this case is to provide the body with enough glucose to increase the intensity of training, but not interrupt ketosis at other times. If you feel tired and lack energy in your training because of a shortage of carbohydrates, then carbohydrate loads before and after can solve this problem. Also, short loads can be better than carbohydrate loading for the entire day. Add 0.5-1 grams of carbohydrates per 1 kilogram of body weight before training. The idea is to use all carbohydrates as fuel to increase the intensity of training. Fats need to be reduced, so that the total caloric content remains unchanged (for fat burning). You can divide the carbohydrates into 2 parts and use one before the workout and the second after.

Cyclical Ketogenic Diet (CKD) includes periodic carbohydrate loads that temporarily refill glycogen reserve in muscles after it is completely depleted. The time between such refills will depend on your goals and intensity of training. Cyclic Keto Diet is an "advanced" option because to understand how often it is best to do carbohydrate loads and how many carbohydrates to consume, you need to try different options and independently determine which one is best for you. After the beginning of ketosis(approximately 2 weeks after the start of the diet) and later once a week, add 5 to 10 grams of carbohydrates per 1 kilogram of dry muscle mass per day. This carbohydrate loading lasts from 9 to 36 hours. Start with 9, and then add 2-4 hours each time and evaluate the results. Note that the amount of protein on such days remains high and fats need to be reduced. If you are on a fat burning diet, then in the days of carbohydrate load calories can be raised to the level of daily norm.

It should be noted that only the basis of the standard keto diet has extensive clinical studies. Cyclical and targeted keto diets are actively practiced by bodybuilding enthusiasts, but their safety is not confirmed clinically, therefore you should consult with your doctor to evaluate your personal health and listen to your body. Start with the standard version of keto diet. After the first few weeks, you can assess how much the intensity of training suffers due to the small amount of carbohydrates. If the trainings are noticeably affected, then you can try a cyclic or targeted keto diet option to add some carbohydrates.

Which option is better for fat burning and which one is good for building muscle mass? The main thing to watch is the number of calories. Excess for muscle growth and a deficit for weight loss (about 500 calories more or less). If the calories match your goals, then keto diet option is not that important. The presence of carbohydrates in pre- and post-training time does help to protect muscles from being lost. Therefore, a cyclic and targeted diet option may be a more appropriate choice for muscle building. But in the long run, periodic carb loads will not have an effect comparable to the effect of the degree of calorie deficit.

Advantages of Keto Diet

Weight Loss
The benefits of keto diet include a quick and effective loss of excess weight, which is supported by studies. The figure on the scale is not reduced by fluid or muscle loss, but by breaking down of fats. You can lose up to 22 pounds a month without feeling hungry.

No feeling of hunger
During the keto diet, you do not have to starve or constantly count calories. Of course, it is necessary to regulate the amount of food consumed, but the keto diet is based not on reducing calories, but on maximizing the minimization of carbohydrate food. You can always grab food from the list of allowed foods.

Long lasting effect
The fact is that most diets for the body are like roller coasters, a constant stress. When nutrients are low, metabolic processes slow down; when they increase- the body cannot cope with processing, and stores excess in form of fat. Keto diet eliminates the appearance of such an effect, since a person does not starve.

Keep muscles
Keto diet does not lead to loss of muscle mass because with keto diet you can get rid of the fat layer while retaining muscles. The weight is lost due to getting rid of subcutaneous and visceral fat and not muscles.

Proven effectiveness
The state of ketosis contributes to a faster loss of body fat compared with other diets, for example, with low fat. This has been proven by numerous studies and personal trials.

Helps with acne
There are a number of reasons for the appearance of acne, and one of them may be the amount of sugar in the blood. Eating foods high in processed and refined carbohydrates can alter the intestinal bacteria and cause sharper fluctuations in blood sugar levels that can affect the health of the skin. Therefore, reducing the carbohydrate intake during ketogenic diet can help get rid some of the types of acne. The low glycemic index of products allowed in keto-diet, also helps improve the skin, prone to acne.

Prevents cancer
A recent study has shown that a ketogenic diet can be an excellent complementary treatment for people with cancer undergoing chemotherapy. This is due to the fact that such a diet causes strong oxidative stress in cancer cells. Other theories suggest that, since a ketogenic diet lowers blood sugar levels, it reduces insulin complications that may be associated with certain cancers.

Potentially reduces seizures
It is believed that the combination of fat, protein and carbohydrates changes the way the body uses energy, which leads to ketosis. Ketosis is an elevated level of ketone bodies in the blood. Ketosis can lead to a reduction in seizures in people with epilepsy. Scientists are still trying to figure out how effective this is in fact, although it is already known that this diet is most effective for children with focal seizures.

Day 2

Cheesy Bacon Brussel Sprouts Casserole (Fat 27.3, Net Carbs 6, Protein 14.2)

Lunch
Beef and Chicken Meatballs (Fat 21 g, Net Carbs 4.3 g, Protein 31.8 g)with Bacon Spinach Salad (Fat 33.9 g, Net Carbs 2.1 g, Protein 12.4 g) and 1 hard boiled egg (Fat 9.64 g, Net Carbs 1.02 g, Protein 8.97 g)

Snack/Dessert
Egg Cream Smoothie (Fat 39.31 g, Net Carbs 3, Protein 21.18 g), Breakfast Egg Muffin (Fat 10 g, Net Carbs 6 g, Protein 14 g)

Dinner
Turkey Taco Casserole (Fat 17.17 g, Net Carbs 4.03 g, Protein 17.59 g)

Day 3

Breakfast

Breakfast Egg Muffin (Fat 10 g, Net Carbs 6 g, Protein 14 g) with ½ avocado, sliced (Fat 14.73 g, Net Carbs 1.87 g, Protein 2.01 g)

Lunch

Cloud Bread (Fat 2.8 g, Net Carbs 0.4 g, Protein 2.2 g) with Chicken and Celery Salad (Fat 19.4 g, Net Carbs 0.4 g, Protein 24.8 g) and ½ avocado, sliced (Fat 14.73 g, Net Carbs 1.87 g, Protein 2.01 g)

Snack/Dessert

Turkey Roll Ups (Fat 5.9 g, Net Carbs 5.38 g, Protein 10.55 g)

Dinner

Fried Chicken Thighs (Fat 20.69 g, Net Carbs 3.49 g, Protein 33.75 g) with Cauliflower "Mac" and Cheese Casserole (Fat 37.73 g, Net Carbs 4.3 g, Protein 18.86 g)and Quail Egg Salad (Fat 30.06 g, Net Carbs 4.56 g, Protein 13.26 g)

Thank you again for reading this book! I really do hope you found the best recipes for you.

If you enjoyed this book I would really appreciate it if you would post a short review on Amazon.com. Your opinion is extremely important for me.

Day 4

Breakfast

Salmon Breakfast Bombs (Fat 23.53 g, Net Carbs 0.96 g, Protein 18.25 g)

Lunch

Sandwich from 2 pieces Cloud Bread (Fat 5.6 g, Net Carbs 0.8 g, Protein 4.4 g), 1 tablespoon pesto, 1 tablespoons cream cheese, 1/3 cup arugula leaves, 2 slices cooked fried bacon (Fat 21.2 g, Net Carbs 1.5 g, Protein 10.6 g)

Snack/Dessert

Cottage Cheese with Walnuts (Fat 34.46 g, Net Carbs 9.84 g, Protein 29.29 g), 2 servings Chocolate Fudge Protein Bars (Fat 29.6 g, Net Carbs 4.2 g, Protein 13.4 g)

Dinner

Comforting Beef Chili (Fat 22.8 g, Net Carbs 5.2 g, Protein 34.4) with Stacked Caprese Salad (Fat 19.3 g, Net Carbs 5.5 g, Protein 11.5 g)

Day 5

Breakfast
Breakfast Egg Roll Ups (Fat 31.66 g, Net Carbs 2.26 g, Protein 28.21 g)

Lunch
Turkey Taco Casserole (Fat 17.17 g, Net Carbs 4.03 g, Protein 17.59 g)

Snack/Dessert
Avocado, Chia Seeds and Cacao Smoothie (Fat 40.1 g, Net Carbs 6.14 g, Protein 35.68 g)

Dinner
Comforting Beef Chili (Fat 22.8 g, Net Carbs 5.2 g, Protein 34.4) with Lebanese Tabbouleh Salad (Fat 45.01 g, Net Carbs 8.52 g, Protein 5.77 g)

Day 6

Breakfast
Easy Banana Bread (Fat 37 g, Net Carbs 4 g, Protein 14 g)

Lunch
Perfect Caesar Salad (Fat 102 g, Net carbs 5 g, Protein 57 g)

Snack/Dessert
2 ounces beef jerky (Fat 14.52 g, Net Carbs 5.24 g, Protein 18.82 g)

Dinner
Juicy Beef with Broccoli (Fat 0.4 g, Net Carbs 4 g, Protein 27 g)with Creamy Garlic Mashed Cauliflower (Fat 10.6 g, Net Carbs 8.28 g, Protein 6.41 g)

Day 7

Breakfast

Greek Yogurt with Nuts and Chia Seeds (Fat 34 g, Net Carbs 6 g, Protein 17 g)

Lunch

Juicy Beef with Broccoli (Fat 0.4 g, Net Carbs 4 g, Protein 27 g)

Snack/Dessert

Peanut Butter Protein Cookies (Fat 6 g, Net Carbs 2 g, Protein 22 g)

Dinner

Avocado Chia Salad (Fat 63.44 g, Net Carbs 10.14 g, Protein 11.47 g) with Simple Chicken Curry (Fat 62 g, Net Carbs 5 g, Protein 39 g)

Day 8

Breakfast

Mini Pizza Egg Bakes (Fat 22.66 g, Net Carbs 4.28 g, Protein 25.59 g) with ½ avocado, sliced (Fat 14.73 g, Net Carbs 1.87 g, Protein 2.01 g)

Lunch

Turkey Taco Casserole (Fat 17.17 g, Net Carbs 4.03 g, Protein 17.59 g)

Snack/Dessert

2 servings Satisfying Cheddar Chips (Fat 18 g, Net Carbs 0 g, Protein 14 g) and 1-2 ounces almonds (Fat 14.36 g, Net Carbs 2.3 g, Protein 6.03 g)

Dinner

Simple Chicken Curry (Fat 62 g, Net Carbs 5 g, Protein 39 g) with Cauliflower Fried Rice with Bacon (Fat 15.94 g, Net Carbs 9.78 g, Protein 9.38 g) topped with ½ cup shredded cheddar cheese (Fat 9 g, Net Carbs 2 g, Protein 7 g)

Day 9

Breakfast

Salmon Breakfast Bombs (Fat 23.53 g, Net Carbs 0:96 g, Protein 18.25 g)

Lunch

Jalapeño Cheddar Stuffed Burger (Fat 52.84 g, Net Carbs 1.6 g, Protein 38.46 g) with Easy Everything Bagels (Fat 35.5 g, Net Carbs 6g, Protein 27.8 g)and ½ avocado (Fat 14.73 g, Net Carbs 1.87 g, Protein 2.01 g)

Snack/Dessert

Avocado Chocolate Pudding (Fat 16.14 g, Net Carbs 5.26 g, Protein 3.96 g)

Dinner

Veggie Mini Meatloaf (Fat 3.5 g, Net Carbs 2.2 g, Protein 21.8 g) with Cauliflower Fried Rice with Bacon (Fat 15.94 g, Net Carbs 9.78 g, Protein 9.38 g)

Day 10

Turkey Sausage Frittata (Fat 16.7, Net Carbs 5.5, Protein 16.7)

Lunch
Jalapeño Cheddar Stuffed Burger (Fat 52.84 g, Net Carbs 1.6 g, Protein 38.46 g), 1 fried egg (Fat 6.83 g, Net Carbs 0.38 g, Protein 6.26 g), 2 ounces cooked spinach (Fat 0.15 g,Net Carbs 0.73 g, Protein 1.68 g)on Easy Everything Bagels (Fat 35.5 g, Net Carbs 6g, Protein 27.8 g)

Snack/Dessert
2 ounces beef jerky (Fat 14.52 g, Net Carbs 5.24 g, Protein 18.82 g) and Peanut Butter Protein Cookies (Fat 6 g, Net Carbs 2 g, Protein 22 g)

Dinner
Cheesy Bacon Brussel Sprouts Casserole (Fat 27.3, Net Carbs 6, Protein 14.2)

Day 11

Easy Banana Bread (Fat 37 g, Net Carbs 4 g, Protein 14 g)

Lunch
Fried Chicken Thighs (Fat 20.69 g, Net Carbs 3.49 g, Protein 33.75 g)with Arugula, Asparagus and Avocado Salad (Fat 48.63 g, Net Carbs 8.71 g, Protein 15.91 g)

Snack/Dessert
2 servings Chocolate Fudge Protein Bars (Fat 29.6 g, Net Carbs 4.2 g, Protein 13.4 g)

Dinner
Beef and Chicken Meatballs (Fat 21 g, Net Carbs 4.3 g Protein 31.8 g) with Quick Zucchini Noodles (Fat 7.28, Net Carbs 0.78 Protein 0.8 g) topped with ½ cup shredded cheddar cheese (Fat 9 g, Net Carbs 2 g, Protein 7 g)

Day 12

Cinnamon Breakfast Pancakes (Fat 45 g, Net Carbs 3.1 g, Protein 19.6 g)

Lunch
Turkey Sausage Frittata (Fat 16.7 g, Net Carbs 5.5 g, Protein 16.7 g)

Snack/Dessert
2 servings Chocolate Fudge Protein Bars (Fat 29.6 g, Net Carbs 4.2 g, Protein 13.4 g)and 1 ounce beef jerky (Fat 7.26 g, Net Carbs 2.62 g, Protein 9.41 g)

Dinner
Bacon Wrapped Chicken Tenders (Fat 38.25 g, Net Carbs 2.7 g, Protein 41.4 g) with Herb Salmon Salad (Fat 21.5 g, Net Carbs 3.5 g, Protein 26.4 g)

Day 13

Breakfast

Easy Banana Bread (Fat 37 g, Net Carbs 4 g, Protein 14 g) withKeto Bulletproof Coffee (Fat 31 g, Net Carbs 0.6 g, Protein 1 g)

Lunch

Bacon Wrapped Chicken Tenders (Fat 38.25 g, Net Carbs 2.7 g, Protein 41.4 g)with Herb Salmon Salad (Fat 21.5 g, Net Carbs 3.5 g, Protein 26.4 g)

Snack/Dessert

Dinner

Cauliflower "Mac" and Cheese Casserole (Fat 37.73 g, Net Carbs 4.3 g, Protein 18.86 g)with Stacked Caprese Salad (Fat 19.3 g, Net Carbs 5.5 g, Protein 11.5 g) and Veggie Mini Meatloaf (Fat 3.5 g, Net Carbs 2.2 g, Protein 21.8 g)

Day 14

Breakfast

Baked Eggs with Cheesy Hash (Fat 18.14 g, Net Carbs 5.77 g, Protein 12.57 g)

Lunch

Jalapeño Cheddar Stuffed Burger (Fat 52.84 g, Net Carbs 1.6 g, Protein 38.46 g) and ½ cup micro greens (Fat 0 g, Net Carbs 0 g, Protein 0.5 g) between 2 pieces Cloud Bread (Fat 5.6 g, Net Carbs 0.8 g, Protein 4.4 g)

Snack/Dessert

1-2 servings No-Bake Protein Bars (Fat 18 g, Net Carbs 1.8 g, Protein 5.3 g for 1 serving)

Dinner

Turkey Taco Casserole (Fat 17.17 g, Net Carbs 4.03 g, Protein 17.59 g) with Lemon Tuna Salad (Fat 40 g, Net Carbs 3 g, Protein 45 g)

Day 15

Breakfast

Easy Banana Bread (Fat 37 g, Net Carbs 4 g, Protein 14 g)

Lunch

Bacon, Avocado, and Chicken Sandwich (Fat 53.25 g, Net Carbs 7.2 g, Protein 43.31 g)

Snack/Dessert

Cottage Cheese with Walnuts (Fat 34.46 g, Net Carbs 9.84 g, Protein 29.29 g), Satisfying Cheddar Chips (Fat 9 g, Net Carbs 0 g, Protein 7 g)

Dinner

Beef and Chicken Meatballs (Fat 21 g, Net Carbs 4.3 g, Protein 31.8 g) with Quick Zucchini Noodles (Fat 7.28, Net Carbs 0.78 Protein 0.8 g)

Day 16

Breakfast

Turkey Sausage Frittata (Fat 16.7 g, Net Carbs 5.5 g, Protein 16.7 g)

Lunch

Perfect Caesar Salad (Fat 102 g, Net carbs 5 g, Protein 57 g)

Snack/Dessert

Moist and Soft Vanilla Cake (Fat 31 g, Net Carbs 2 g, Protein 9 g) and No-Bake Protein Bars (Fat 18 g, Net Carbs 1.8 g, Protein 5.3 g)

Dinner

Juicy Beef with Broccoli (Fat 0.4 g, Net Carbs 4 g, Protein 27 g) with Creamy Garlic Mashed Cauliflower (Fat 10.6 g, Net Carbs 8.28 g, Protein 6.41 g)

Day 17

Breakfast

Cheesy Bacon Brussel Sprouts Casserole (Fat 27.3, Net Carbs 6, Protein 14.2)

Lunch

Coleslaw-Stuffed Wraps (Fat 59.8 g, Net Carbs 5.1 g, Protein 40.14 g)

Snack/Dessert

Moist and Soft Vanilla Cake (Fat 31 g, Net Carbs 2 g, Protein 9 g), Avocado, Chia Seeds and Cacao Smoothie (Fat 40.1 g, Net Carbs 6.14 g, Protein 35.68 g)

Dinner

Juicy Beef with Broccoli (Fat 0.4 g, Net Carbs 4 g, Protein 27 g) with Quick Zucchini Noodles (Fat 7.28, Net Carbs 0.78 Protein 0.8 g)

Day 18

Breakfast

Turkey Sausage Frittata (Fat 16.7, Net Carbs 5.5, Protein 16.7), Peanut Butter Protein Cookies (Fat 6 g, Net Carbs 2 g, Protein 22 g) with Keto Bulletproof Coffee (Fat 31 g, Net Carbs 0.6 g, Protein 1 g)

Lunch

Coleslaw-Stuffed Wraps (Fat 59.8 g, Net Carbs 5.1 g, Protein 40.14 g)

Snack/Dessert

2 servings Chocolate Fudge Protein Bars (Fat 29.6 g, Net Carbs 4.2 g, Protein 13.4 g)

Dinner

Veggie Mini Meatloaf (Fat 3.5 g, Net Carbs 2.2 g, Protein 21.8 g) with Creamy Garlic Mashed Cauliflower (Fat 10.6 g, Net Carbs 8.28 g, Protein 6.41 g)

Day 19

Breakfast

Easy Banana Bread (Fat 37 g, Net Carbs 4 g, Protein 14 g) withKeto Bulletproof Coffee (Fat 31 g, Net Carbs 0.6 g, Protein 1 g)

Lunch

Turkey Roll Ups (Fat 5.9 g, Net Carbs 5.38 g, Protein 10.55 g)

Snack/Dessert

Moist and Soft Vanilla Cake (Fat 31 g, Net Carbs 2 g, Protein 9 g)

Dinner

Spinach Stuffed Chicken Breast (Fat 46.98 g, Net Carbs 2.8 g, Protein 64.51 g) with Herb Salmon Salad (Fat 21.5 g, Net Carbs 3.5 g, Protein 26.4 g)

Day 20

Breakfast

Cinnamon Breakfast Pancakes (Fat 45 g, Net Carbs 3.1 g, Protein 19.6 g) and Egg Cream Smoothie (Fat 39.31 g, Net Carbs 3, Protein 21.18 g)

Lunch

Herb Salmon Salad (Fat 21.5 g, Net Carbs 3.5 g, Protein 26.4 g)

Snack/Dessert

1 ounce almonds (Fat 14.36 g, Net Carbs 2.3 g, Protein 6.03 g)

Dinner

Cauliflower "Mac" and Cheese Casserole (Fat 37.73 g, Net Carbs 4.3 g, Protein 18.86 g) with Fried Chicken Thighs (Fat 20.69 g, Net Carbs 3.49 g, Protein 33.75 g)

Day 21

Breakfast

Avocado Breakfast Bowl (Fat 40 g, Net Carbs 3 g, Protein 25 g)

Lunch

Bacon Spinach Salad (Fat 33.9 g, Net Carbs 2.1 g, Protein 12.4 g) and 1 hard-boiled egg (Fat 9.64 g, Net Carbs 1.02 g, Protein 8.97 g)

Snack/Dessert

Avocado, Chia Seeds and Cacao Smoothie (Fat 40.1 g, Net Carbs 6.14 g, Protein 35.68 g)

Dinner

Veggie Mini Meatloaf (Fat 3.5 g, Net Carbs 2.2 g, Protein 21.8 g)with Creamy Garlic Mashed Cauliflower (Fat 10.6 g, Net Carbs 8.28 g, Protein 6.41 g) and Quail Egg Salad (Fat 30.06 g, Net Carbs 4.56 g, Protein 13.26 g)

Day 22

Breakfast
Mini Pizza Egg Bakes (Fat 22.66 g, Net Carbs 4.28 g, Protein 25.59 g)

Lunch
Comforting Beef Chili (Fat 22.8 g, Net Carbs 5.2 g, Protein 34.4)with Avocado Chia Salad
(Fat 63.44 g, Net Carbs 10.14 g, Protein 11.47 g)

Snack/Dessert
Satisfying Cheddar Chips (Fat 9 g, Net Carbs 0 g, Protein 7 g)

Dinner
Beef and Chicken Meatballs (Fat 21 g, Net Carbs 4.3 g, Protein 31.8 g) with Bacon
Spinach Salad (Fat 33.9 g, Net Carbs 2.1 g, Protein 12.4 g)

Day 23

Breakfast

Easy Banana Bread (Fat 37 g, Net Carbs 4 g, Protein 14 g)

Lunch

Bacon, Avocado, and Chicken Sandwich (Fat 53.25 g, Net Carbs 7.2 g, Protein 43.31 g) and 1 hard-boiled egg (Fat 9.64 g, Net Carbs 1.02 g, Protein 8.97 g)

Snack/Dessert

Cottage Cheese with Walnuts (Fat 34.46 g, Net Carbs 9.84 g, Protein 29.29 g)

Dinner

Cloud Bread (Fat 2.8 g, Net Carbs 0.4 g, Protein 2.2 g) with Chicken and Celery Salad (Fat 19.4 g, Net Carbs 0.4 g, Protein 24.8 g) and ½ avocado, sliced (Fat 14.73 g, Net Carbs 1.87 g, Protein 2.01 g)

Day 24

Breakfast Egg Muffin (Fat 10 g, Net Carbs 6 g, Protein 14 g)

Lunch
Jalapeño Cheddar Stuffed Burger (Fat 52.84 g, Net Carbs 1.6 g, Protein 38.46 g) and ½ cup micro greens (Fat 0 g, Net Carbs 0 g, Protein 0.5 g) between 2 pieces Cloud Bread (Fat 5.6 g, Net Carbs 0.8 g, Protein 4.4 g)

Snack/Dessert
1 ounce beef jerky (Fat 7.26 g, Net Carbs 2.62 g, Protein 9.41 g)

Dinner
Bacon Wrapped Chicken Tenders (Fat 38.25 g, Net Carbs 2.7 g, Protein 41.4 g) with Mixed Green Spring Salad (Fat 42.37 g, Net Carbs 4.88 g, Protein 20.07 g)

Day 25

Breakfast

Egg Benedict with Hollandaise Sauce (Fat 36.9 g, Net Carbs 2.8 g, Protein 30.5 g)

Lunch

Bacon Wrapped Chicken Tenders (Fat 38.25 g, Net Carbs 2.7 g, Protein 41.4 g)with Quick Zucchini Noodles (Fat 7.28, Net Carbs 0.78 Protein 0.8 g)

Snack/Dessert

Breakfast Egg Muffin (Fat 10 g, Net Carbs 6 g, Protein 14 g)

Dinner

Cauliflower "Mac" and Cheese Casserole (Fat 37.73 g, Net Carbs 4.3 g, Protein 18.86 g)with Chicken and Celery Salad (Fat 19.4 g, Net Carbs 0.4 g, Protein 24.8 g)

Day 26

Mini Pizza Egg Bakes (Fat 22.66 g, Net Carbs 4.28 g, Protein 25.59 g)

Lunch
Perfect Caesar Salad (Fat 102 g, Net carbs 5 g, Protein 57 g)

Snack/Dessert
Turkey Roll Ups (Fat 5.9 g, Net Carbs 5.38 g, Protein 10.55 g)

Dinner
Veggie Mini Meatloaf (Fat 3.5 g, Net Carbs 2.2 g, Protein 21.8 g) with Cauliflower Fried Rice with Bacon (Fat 15.94 g, Net Carbs 9.78 g, Protein 9.38 g)

Day 27

Breakfast

Salmon Breakfast Bombs (Fat 23.53 g, Net Carbs 0.96 g, Protein 18.25 g)

Lunch

Herb Salmon Salad (Fat 21.5 g, Net Carbs 3.5 g, Protein 26.4 g)
and 1 hard-boiled egg (Fat 9.64 g, Net Carbs 1.02 g, Protein 8.97 g)

Snack/Dessert

Moist and Soft Vanilla Cake (Fat 31 g, Net Carbs 2 g, Protein 9 g)

Dinner

Simple Chicken Curry (Fat 62 g, Net Carbs 5 g, Protein 39 g) with Cauliflower Fried Rice with Bacon (Fat 15.94 g, Net Carbs 9.78 g, Protein 9.38 g) topped with ½ cup shredded cheddar cheese (Fat 9 g, Net Carbs 2 g, Protein 7 g)

Day 28

Breakfast
Breakfast Egg Roll Ups (Fat 31.66 g, Net Carbs 2.26 g, Protein 28.21 g)

Lunch
Coloslaw-Stuffed Wraps (Fat 59.8 g, Net Carbs 5.1 g, Protein 40.14 g)

Snack/Dessert
Peanut Butter Protein Cookies (Fat 6 g, Net Carbs 2 g, Protein 22 g)

Dinner
Simple Chicken Curry (Fat 62 g, Net Carbs 5 g, Protein 39 g) with Cloud Bread (Fat 2.8 g, Net Carbs 0.4 g, Protein 2.2 g)

Day 29

Breakfast
Egg Benedict with Hollandaise Sauce (Fat 36.9 g, Net Carbs 2.8 g, Protein 30.5 g)

Lunch
Coleslaw-Stuffed Wraps (Fat 59.8 g, Net Carbs 5.1 g, Protein 40.14 g)

Snack/Dessert
Moist and Soft Vanilla Cake (Fat 31 g, Net Carbs 2 g, Protein 9 g)

Dinner
Chicken and Celery Salad (Fat 19.4 g, Net Carbs 0.4 g, Protein 24.8 g) with Cloud Bread (Fat 2.8 g, Net Carbs 0.4 g, Protein 2.2 g) and 1 hard-boiled egg (Fat 9.64 g, Net Carbs 1.02 g, Protein 8.97 g)

Day 30

Greek Yogurt with Nuts and Chia Seeds (Fat 34 g, Net Carbs 6 g, Protein 17 g)

Lunch
Chicken and Celery Salad (Fat 19.4 g, Net Carbs 0.4 g, Protein 24.8 g) with Cloud Bread (Fat 2.8 g, Net Carbs 0.4 g, Protein 2.2 g)

Snack/Dessert
Moist and Soft Vanilla Cake (Fat 31 g, Net Carbs 2 g, Protein 9 g) with Keto Bulletproof Coffee (Fat 31 g, Net Carbs 0.6 g, Protein 1 g)

Dinner
Veggie Mini Meatloaf (Fat 3.5 g, Net Carbs 2.2 g, Protein 21.8 g) with Lemon Tuna Salad (Fat 40 g, Net Carbs 3 g, Protein 45 g)

Recipes. Simple and Easy Breakfast. Egg Benedict
with Hollandaise Sauce

Ingredients (1 serving):
Eggs Benedict:

- 1 cloud bread (see Easy Cloud Bread)
- 2 eggs
- 2 slices bacon
- ½ tablespoon white vinegar
- ½ teaspoon chives

Hollandaise sauce:

- 1 egg yolks
- 1 tablespoon butter
- ½ tablespoon lemon juice
- Pinch salt
- Pinch paprika

Instructions:

1. Prepare cloud bread according to the instructions (see Easy Cloud Bread) or use leftovers.
2. Separate the egg for the sauce and place in heat proof bowl. Whisk yolk until doubled in size, thenwhisk in lemon juice.
3. Add about an inch of water to a pot and bring to simmer. Meanwhile, melt butter in microwave for 30 to 60 seconds, until melted.
4. Place a bowl with egg yolk on top of the pot without the bottom touching the water (make a double boiler) and whisk egg yolk until they start to thicken.
5. Remove from heat and slowly whisk in melted butter. Return on top of the pot and let the sauce thicken more until it coats a spoon when lifted out.
6. Remove sauce from heat and set aside. Add salt and paprika to taste and if it gets too thick, whisk in a little water.
7. Add about 3 inches of water to a pot and bring to boil. Reduce heat to simmering and stir in some salt and white vinegar.
8. Carefully crack the egg into a cup. Stir the water in around in one direction to make a whirlpool, then lower the cup and gently slide the egg into the whirlpool. Cook for 2 to 4 minutes and carefully remove with a spatula onto a plate lined with paper towel. Repeat with the second egg.
9. If desired, fry the bacon in a pan until crispy and warm. Slice cloud bread in half and place each slice on top of the cut side of each piece. Add poached eggs on top of each slice of bacon and finish with a spoonful of hollandaise sauce and chopped chives.
10. Serve.

Salmon Breakfast Bombs

Ingredients (1 serving):
Breakfast bombs

- 1 large egg
- 2 ounces smoked salmon slices
- 1 teaspoon salted butter
- 1 tablespoon fresh chives, chopped
- Salt and pepper to taste

Hollandaise sauce:

- 1 tablespoons salted butter, room temperature
- 1 large egg yolk, separated from the white
- 1/8 teaspoon Dijon mustard
- 1 teaspoon lemon juice, freshly squeezed
- 1/2 teaspoon water, add more if too thick
- Salt to taste

Instructions:

1. Bring a small pot of water to boil. Carefully add the egg and cook for 10 to 12 minutes. Meanwhile, chop fresh chives and finely dice salmon slices. When egg is cooked, place it in cold water to cool. Peel and finely mash with a fork.
2. Heat 1 teaspoon butter in a pan over high heat. Add half of the salmon and cook until crispy. Set aside.
3. Add 1 or 2 cups of water to a pot and bring to simmer on the stovetop.
4. Add 1 tablespoon butter to a bowl and melt in microwave for 30 to 60 seconds, until melted but not hot. Set aside.
5. Add egg yolk, lemon juice, Dijon mustard and a pinch of salt to a heat-safe bowl and whisk until air bubbles appear.
6. Place the bowl with egg mixture on top of the pot with simmering water, without have the water touch the bowl. Cook, continuously whisking, until it starts to thicken.
7. When the egg mixture starts to thicken, remove the bowl from the pot and slowly whisk in melted butter. Return the bowl onto the pot and cook until the sauce is fully thickened. Add a little water to thin it out, if desired. Remove and allow to cool to room temperature.
8. Add raw salmon, half of the chives to the egg and stir in hollandaise (not all at once), until well combined. Do not use all sauce if the mixture starts to get too wet and is not firm.
9. Roll the mixture into four balls and then roll in a mixture of crispy salmon and reserved chives.
10. Enjoy! Store in refrigerator for up to 3 days.

Greek Yogurt with Nuts and Chia Seeds

Ingredients (1 serving):

- ½ cup full fat Greek yogurt
- 1/3 cup or more vanilla unsweetened almond milk
- ¼ cup pecans or other nuts
- 1 tablespoon chia seeds
- ½ tablespoon no-sugar added vanilla syrup or another sweetener to taste

Instructions:

1. Add yogurt, milk and sweetener to a bowl and stir until well combined and smooth.
2. Stir chia seeds and, if desired, refrigerate for about 10 minutes for thicker consistency.
3. Top with chopped pecans or other nuts of your choice.
4. Serve.

Cinnamon Breakfast Pancakes

Ingredients (1 serving):

- ¼ cup plus ½ tablespoon almond or coconut flour
- ¼ cup cream cheese
- 2 eggs
- ¼ teaspoon cinnamon
- ½ tablespoon butter or avocado oil, for frying
- 1 teaspoon butter, for serving

Instructions:

1. Add flour, cream cheese, and eggs to a blender and blend until well combined and no lumps remain.
2. Heat butter or avocado oil in a frying pan over medium heat.
3. Once hot, add 2 to 3 tablespoons batter to make a pancake and cook for 3 to 4 minutes or until bubbles appear in the center and then flip and cook on the other side. Repeat with the remaining batter to make a total of 2 to 3 pancakes.
4. Sprinkle with cinnamon and top with butter.
5. Enjoy!

Mini Pizza Egg Bakes

Ingredients (1 serving):

- 3 large eggs, separated
- 4 tablespoons shredded mozzarella cheese
- 1 teaspoons Italian herb blend
- 2 large black olives, sliced
- 4 large mild pepper rings
- 1 tablespoon diced red bell pepper
- 1 tablespoon tomato sauce

Instructions:

1. Add 1 tablespoons mozzarella cheese and Italian herb blend to a microwave or oven save dish.
2. Separate eggs and beat egg whites just to break them and combine. Add to the cheese in the bowl and microwave for 1 ½ to 2 minutes, until egg whites are set. Set aside to cool.
3. Slice black olives and dice bell pepper. Beat egg yolks and lightly scramble on a skillet.
4. Add black olives, pepper rings, bell pepper and ½ tablespoon tomato sauce to the egg yolk and fold into the egg. Set aside.
5. Top egg white with reserved tomato sauce and then scrambled egg mixture. Sprinkle with remaining mozzarella cheese and microwave for 20 seconds or broil until the cheese has melted and is bubbly.
6. Serve hot.

Breakfast Egg Muffins

Ingredients (2 servings):

- 1/2 teaspoon salt
- 1/4 teaspoon organic coconut oil
- 1/2 cup broccoli, chopped
- 1/4 onion, chopped
- 1/8 whole green bell pepper, chopped
- 1/8 whole red bell pepper, chopped
- 1/2 teaspoon black pepper
- 4 pastured eggs
- 1 teaspoon primal palate adobo seasoning, (or 1 teaspoon salt, 1 teaspoon pepper)

Instructions:

1. Preheat oven to 400°F. Grease a small muffin tin or 2 oven safe cups with coconut oil.
2. Chop broccoli, onion, and green and red bell pepper into 1/3-inch pieces. Divide between 2 muffin tins.
3. Add eggs to a bowl and whisk together. Add to the vegetables, dividing evenly.
4. Season eggs and vegetables with salt and pepper and stir together. Bake for 18 to 20 minutes.
5. Flip egg muffins onto a serving plate.
6. Serve right away or refrigerate for up to 4 days.

Turkey Sausage Frittata

Ingredients (4 servings):

- 6 ounces ground breakfast sausage, turkey
- 1 bell peppers, sliced into strips
- 6 eggs
- 1/2 cup lactose free sour cream
- ½ teaspoon pink Himalayan salt
- ½ teaspoon black pepper
- 1 teaspoon butter
- 2 ounces shredded Tillamook cheddar optional

Instructions:

1. Preheat the oven to 350°F. Cut bell pepper into strips.
2. Place eggs, sour cream, salt and pepper into a blender and blend for 30 seconds on high. Set aside.
3. Place a large skillet over medium heat and add butter when hot. Add bell pepper and cook until tender and browned, about 6 minutes. Transfer the pepper to a plate.
4. Add turkey sausage and cook, breaking up, for about 8 minutes or until browned.
5. Flatten the sausage on the bottom and add a layer of peppers. Top with egg mixture.
6. Transfer the skillet into an oven and bake for 30 minutes. If using cheese, sprinkle it over the frittata as soon as you take it out. Allow the cheese to melt before slicing.
7. Serve. Allow to cool completely, then cut into portion sizes and freeze for 2 to 3 months. Allow to thaw in refrigerator overnight before reheating in the oven or microwave.

Breakfast Egg Roll Ups

Ingredients (1 serving):

- 2 large eggs
- Salt and pepper to taste
- 1/3 cup shredded cheddar cheese
- 1 slicebacon, cooked
- 1 patty breakfast sausage, cooked

Instructions:

1. Heat a non-stick skillet over medium heat. Meanwhile, whisk the eggs together in a bowl and then pour into the skillet. Add salt and pepper to taste and cook, covered, over medium low heat for a few minutes or until the eggs are almost set.
2. Evenly spread cheddar cheese over the eggs and top with a slice of bacon. Break a sausage patty in half and place on top the bacon. Carefully roll the eggs so it is folded about in thirds. Let the egg set and transfer on a serving plate.
3. Serve hot.

Cottage Cheese with Walnuts

Ingredients (1 serving):
- 1 cup cottage cheese
- 1 handful of walnuts, chopped
- Dash of cinnamon
- Sprinkle of salt

Instructions:
1. Chop walnuts.
2. Place cottage cheese into a bowl, if desired, or leave in a container.
3. Top with walnuts and sprinkle with cinnamon and salt to taste.
4. Enjoy!

Cheesy Bacon Brussel Sprouts Casserole

Ingredients (3 servings):

- 4 slices bacon, cut into strips
- 1/2 fresh brussels sprouts, washed, dried, quartered
- 1 tablespoon avocado oil
- Salt and pepper
- Avocado oil cooking spray
- 1/2 small yellow onion, diced
- ½ tablespoon minced garlic
- 1/2 cup grated parmesan
- 1 ounce shredded sharp cheddar
- 1/3 cup heavy whipping cream
- Pinch nutmeg

Instructions:

1. Preheat the oven to 375°F. Line a baking sheet with aluminum foil.
2. Wash, dry and quarter brussels sprouts and place into a mixing bowl. Add avocado oil, salt and pepper and toss together.
3. Transfer brussels sprouts into a baking sheet and bake for 15 minutes.
4. Meanwhile, heat a skillet and add bacon strips. Cook until crisp and transfer using a slotted spoon onto paper towels. Keep the grease in the skillet.
5. Dice onion and mince garlic. Place into the skillet with the grease from bacon and cook, stirring often, until aromatic.
6. Return bacon to the skillet and cook until heated through. Remove from heat.
7. Place parmesan cheese, cheddar cheese, heavy whipping cream, nutmeg, salt and pepper into a bowl and whisk together.
8. Grease a casserole dish and add brussels sprouts and bacon mixture. Mix everything together.
9. Pour the egg and cheese mixture over brussels sprouts. Bake for 15 minutes, then broil for 2 minutes or until the cheese is golden brown. Allow to cool before serving.
10. Serve and freeze leftovers in individual portions.

Avocado Breakfast Bowl

Ingredients (1 serving):

- 1 avocado, halved and the stone removed
- 1 tbsp salted butter
- 3 large eggs
- 3 rashers of bacon, cut into small pieces
- Pinch of salt and black pepper

Instructions:

1. Scoop out most of the flesh from the avocado.
2. Add butter to a large saucepan and melt over low heat. Meanwhile, beat together eggs with salt and pepper in a separate bowl.
3. Add bacon to one side of the saucepan and fry for 2 to 3 minutes. Pour eggs on the other side and scramble, stirring often, for about 5 minutes more.
4. Stir the eggs and bacon together and add to the avocado shells.
5. Serve.

Keto Bulletproof Coffee

Ingredients (8 ounces):

- 1 cup freshly brewed hot coffee
- 1 tablespoon grass fed butter
- 1/2 scoop MCT oil powder
- 1/2 teaspoon ceylon cinnamon

Instructions:

1. Brew fresh coffee.
2. Add hot coffee, butter, MCT oil powder and Ceylon cinnamon to a blender and blend on low for 30 seconds or until frothy.
3. Pour bulletproof coffee into a cup.
4. Enjoy!

Baked Eggs with Cheesy Hash

Ingredients (1 serving):

- 1 1/2 ounces zucchini, diced
- 2 ounces chopped cauliflower
- ¼ medium red bell pepper, diced
- 1/3 tablespoon coconut oil, melted
- 1/3 teaspoon smoked paprika
- 1/3 teaspoon onion powder
- 1/4 teaspoon garlic powder
- 2/3 ounce Mexican blend shredded cheese
- 1/4 medium avocado, sliced
- 1 large egg
- 1/3 tablespoon sliced jalapenos, optional
- 1 tablespoon cotija cheese
- 2/3 teaspoon Tajín seasoning

Instructions:

1. Preheat the oven to 400°F. Line a small baking sheet/pan with foil.
2. Dice zucchini, chop cauliflower, and dice bell pepper.
3. Add zucchini, cauliflower and red bell pepper to the pan. Drizzle with oil and sprinkle with onion powder, garlic powder and paprika. Toss everything and spread into a single layer.
4. Bake for 10 to 15 minutes or until the vegetables start to brown.
5. Meanwhile, slice avocado. Take out the vegetables and sprinkle with shredded cheese. Top with avocado slices and crack an egg over the vegetables.
6. Bake for 10 minutes longer or until the egg is cooked to desired doneness.
7. Serve topped with cotija cheese, jalapenos, if desired, and Tajin seasoning.

Satisfying Main Dishes. Coleslaw-Stuffed Wraps

Ingredients (2 servings):
Coleslaw:

- 1 ½ cups thinly sliced red cabbage
- 1/4 cup diced green onions
- 1/3 cup mayonnaise
- 1 teaspoon apple cider vinegar
- Finely groundsea salt to taste

Wraps and additional filling:

- 8 collard leaves, stems removed
- ½ pound regular ground meat (beef, chicken, pork or turkey), cooked and chilled
- ½ ounce alfalfa sprouts
- 1 cup cheddar cheese
- Toothpicks, for holding the wraps together

Instructions:

1. Thinly slice red cabbage and dice green onions. Add mayonnaise, apple cider vinegar and salt to taste and mix until well combined.
2. Cut out the stem from collard leaves from about midway of the leaf.
3. Add a spoonful of cooked ground meat to the end that is not cut and top with slaw mixture alfalfa sprouts and cheddar cheese, dividing everything evenly among all the leaves.
4. Roll starting from the end with a filling and tuck the sides as you go. Secure with 1 or 2 toothpicks.
5. Serve and refrigerate leftovers in an airtight container.

Spinach Stuffed Chicken Breasts

Ingredients (2 servings):

- 2 chicken breasts
- 1/2 tablespoon olive oil
- 1/2 teaspoon paprika
- 1/2 teaspoon salt divided
- ¼ teaspoon garlic powder
- ¼ teaspoon onion powder
- 2 ounces cream cheese, softened
- 1/8 cup grated Parmesan
- 1 tablespoon mayonnaise
- 3/4 cup chopped fresh spinach
- 1/2 teaspoon garlic, minced
- 1/4 teaspoon red pepper flakes

Instructions:

1. Preheat the oven to 375°F.
2. In a small bowl stir together ¼ teaspoon salt, garlic powder, and onion powder.
3. Place chicken breasts onto a cutting board. Drizzle with olive oil and sprinkle with salt mixture on both sides.
4. Make a pocket cutting horizontally into the side of the chicken breast. Set aside.
5. In a small bowl combine well together cream cheese, parmesan cheese, mayonnaise, spinach, garlic, red pepper and remaining salt.
6. Divide spinach and cheese mixture between the two breasts, adding it into the pocket.
7. Set chicken breasts on a baking sheet/dish and bake for 25 minutes, or until the chicken breasts are cooked through.
8. Serve.

Veggie Mini Meatloafs

Ingredients (6 servings):

- 1 poundground beef or pork
- 3/4 teaspoon sea salt
- 1/2 teaspoon ground black pepper
- 1 large egg
- 1/2 medium onion, finely chopped
- 1 cup mushrooms,finely chopped
- 1/4 cup fincly chopped or grated carrots
- 1 loosely packed cup spinach, finely chopped
- 1/2 teaspoon dry thyme
- 2 cloves garlic, minced

Instructions:

1. Preheat the oven to 350°F. Grease a 6-hole muffin tin.
2. Finely chop onion, mushrooms and spinach and grate or finely chop carrot. Mince garlic.
3. Place ground meat, salt, black pepper, egg, onion, mushrooms, carrots, spinach, thyme, and garlic. Mix everything with clean hands until well combined together.
4. Divide the meat mixture among the 6 muffin holes. Bake for 25 to 30 minutes, until meat is cooked through.
5. Serve right away and freeze leftovers or store in fridge for up to 5 days.

Jalapeño Cheddar Stuffed Burger

Ingredients (4 servings):
- 28 ounces ground beef (80/20)
- 2 tablespoons finely minced onion
- Salt & pepper to taste
- 4 tablespoons cream cheese
- 2 ounces shredded cheddar cheese
- 1/4 teaspoon garlic powder
- 1 fresh jalapeno pepper, diced (seeds removed for less spice)
- 1 tablespoon olive oil
- Rolls and toppings as desired

Instructions:
1. Finely mince onion and dice jalapeno pepper.
2. Preheat grill to medium or oven to broil on high.
3. Add cream cheese, cheddar cheese, garlic powder and jalapeno pepper and mix together. Make 4 patties from cheese mixture.
4. In another bowl, combine ground beef with onion and season with salt and pepper. Divide the meat mixture into 4 and wrap around cheese patties.
5. Lightly brush each burger with olive oil.
6. Grill burgers for 6 to 7 minutes per side, until cooked through (internal temperature of 160°F). Alternatively, place on a pan lined with foil and broil in the oven about 6 inches away from the broiler for 5 to 6 minutes per side, or until cooked through.
7. Serve as desired. Refrigerate leftover within 1 to 2 hours of cooking or freeze in individual freezer bags for 2 to 6 months. Let them thaw in the refrigerator for a few hours or reheat them from frozen.

Bacon Wrapped Chicken Tenders

Ingredients (2 servings):

- 1 teaspoon kosher salt
- 1 teaspoon ground cayenne pepper (reduce for less spice)
- 1 teaspoon paprika
- 1 teaspoon garlic powder
- 1/2 teaspoon onion powder
- 1/2 teaspoon oregano
- 1/2 teaspoon thyme
- 12 ounces (3/4 pound) chicken tenders (about 6 tenders)
- 6 slices no sugar bacon

Instructions:

1. Preheat oven to 425°F. Line a rimmed baking sheet with aluminum foil and place a metal rack on top.
2. Add salt, cayenne pepper, paprika, garlic powder, onion powder, oregano and thyme to a large zipper bag and shake to mix together.
3. Add 1 chicken tender to the bag and shake to coat in spices. Remove from the bag and wrap in a piece of bacon. Set on a rack, tucking the bacon end, and repeat for the remaining chicken tenders.
4. Place into the oven and bake for 35 minutes. If bacon is not crispy, turn on the broiler and broil for 1 to 2 minutes.
5. Serve.

Simple Chicken Curry

Ingredients (2 servings):
- ¼ tablespoon coconut oil or oil of your choice
- 2 chicken thighs, boneless skinless, cut into 1" pieces
- 1/4 large onion,cut into large chunks
- ½ cup button mushrooms, quartered
- 1/2 small zucchini,cut in half lengthwise and thickly sliced
- 1/4 teaspoon garlic,minced
- 1/8 tablespoon curry powder
- Pinch paprika
- 1/2 teaspoon salt
- 4 ounces canned coconut milk
- Cilantro (to garnish)

Instructions:
1. Cut chicken thighs into 1-inch pieces. Cut onion into large chunks, quarter mushrooms, cut zucchini in half lengthwise and then into thick slices and mince garlic.
2. Add oil to a stock pot and heat over high heat. Add chicken pieces and brown on both sides. Remove onto a plate and save the oil in the pot.
3. Add onion, zucchini and mushrooms to the pot and sauté until lightly browned. Stir in garlic, curry powder, paprika and salt and cook for 30 seconds.
4. Return chicken to the pot and stir in coconut milk. Bring to boil and then lower the heat and simmer, covered, for ½ hour or until chicken is cooked through and tender.
5. Serve chicken with coconut broth garnished with cilantro.

Juicy Beef with Broccoli

Ingredients (2 servings):

- 1/2pound beef (sirloin, skirt steak, boneless short ribs…etc.)
- ½ to 1 heads broccoli, break into florets
- 1 clove garlic, minced
- 1 piece thin sliced ginger, finely chopped
- Ghee or cooking fat of your choice

Beef marinade:

- 1tablespoon coconut aminos
- 1/4 teaspoon coarse sea salt
- 1/2tablespoon sesame oil
- 1/8 teaspoon black pepper
- 1/2 teaspoon arrowroot/sweet potato powder
- 1/8 teaspoon baking soda

Sauce combo:

- 1 tablespoons coconut aminos
- 1/2 tablespoon fish sauce
- 1 teaspoon sesame oil
- 1/8 teaspoon black pepper

Instructions:

1. Prepare marinade by mixing together coconut aminos, sea salt, sesame oil, black pepper arrowroot powder and baking soda.
2. Cut beef into 1/4-inch-thick slices and place into the marinade mixture. Stir to coat and set aside to marinade (refrigerate, if not cooking right away).
3. Brake broccoli into florets and place in a microwave safe bowl. Add 1 to 2 tablespoons water and loosely cover with a lid. Cook in microwave for 2 minutes or until tender, but still crunchy.
4. Add about 1 tablespoon ghee or other fat of choice to a wok and heat over medium heat.
5. Meanwhile, mince garlic and ginger. Add both to the wok, when hot, and reduce heat to medium. Add a pinch of salt and stir fry for 10 seconds or until aromatic.
6. Increase heat to medium high and add marinated beef and spread it in an even layer. Cook beef until the edges start to brown and get crispy, then flip and cook the other side until the meat is about 3 /4 way cooked through and is browned and crispy on the outside.
7. Stir in sauce ingredients (coconut aminos, fish sauce, sesame oil and black pepper) and stir fry for 1 minute. Add broccoli florets and stir fry for about 30 seconds. Toss to mix everything together.
8. Serve.

Turkey Taco Casserole

Ingredients (4 servings):
- ½ pound ground turkey
- ½ small cauliflower, chopped
- ½ jalapeno, chopped
- 1/8 cup chopped red peppers
- 1/8 cup chopped onion
- ½ teaspoon cumin
- ½ teaspoon parsley
- ½ teaspoon turmeric
- ½ teaspoon minced garlic
- ½ teaspoon oregano
- ¾ cup shredded cheddar cheese
- ½ cup sour cream

Instructions:
1. Chop cauliflower, jalapeno, red peppers, and onion and mince garlic.
2. Add ground turkey, cauliflower, cumin, parsley, turmeric, garlic, and oregano to a bowl and mix to combine.
3. Add onion, red peppers and jalapenos and mix together.
4. Stir in ½ cup shredded cheddar cheese and transfer the mixture into a casserole dish. Sprinkle remaining cheese on top.
5. Bake at 350°F for 1 hour. Remove and let cool slightly before cutting.
6. Serve with sour cream. Freeze leftovers in individual portions and reheat in the oven or microwave.

Comforting Beef Chili

Ingredients (3 servings):

- ¼ tablespoon avocado oil
- 1 rib celery, chopped
- 1 pound 85/15 ground beef
- ½ teaspoon ground chipotle chili powder
- ½ tablespoon chili powder
- 1 teaspoon garlic powder
- 1/2 tablespoon cumin
- ½ teaspoon salt
- ½ teaspoon black pepper
- ½ ounce no-salt-added tomato sauce
- ½ ounce beef bone broth
- Optional garnishes: sour cream, cheddar cheese, sliced jalapeno, cilantro, green onion

Instructions:

1. Add avocado oil to a large pot and heat over medium heat. Chop celery and add to the pot. Cook for 3 to 4 minutes, until softened. Transfer celery to a bowl and set aside.
2. Add beef, chipotle chili powder, chili powder, garlic powder, cumin, salt and pepper to the same pot and cook, breaking up meat, until the meat is browned and cooked through.
3. Reduce heat to medium low and stir in tomato sauce and beef bone broth. Simmer, covered, for 10 minutes stirring from time to time.
4. Return celery to the pot and stir to combine.
5. Serve with garnishes of your choice and freeze leftovers in individual portions.

Fried Chicken Thighs

Ingredients (4 servings):

- 4 boneless, skinless chicken thighs or other cuts of chicken totaling 1 pound
- 3 ounces pork rinds
- 3/4 cup parmesan cheese
- 1 egg
- 1/8 cup hot sauce
- 1 tablespoon Italian herb blend
- Oil for frying
- Ranch or other sauce for dipping (optional)

Instructions:

1. Add egg and hot sauce in a large bowl and beat together. Season with salt and pepper.
2. Place chicken into the egg mixture and toss to coat. Refrigerate for at least 1 hour or overnight.
3. Add pork rinds, parmesan cheese, Italian seasoning to a blender and pulse until very fine, almost dust like. Transfer to a large bowl.
4. Add about 1/3 inch of oil to a heavy frying pan (or deep fryer) and heat until hot.
5. Meanwhile, dip chicken thigh one at a time into egg mixture (let excess drip), then coat in "breading" mixture and add to the pan. Repeat with remaining chicken breasts, but do not overcrowd the frying pan.
6. Cook for 4 minutes, then 4 minutes or until cooked through (165°F internal temperature) on the other side. If necessary, flip couple more times to prevent breading from burning. Alternatively, transfer on a lined baking sheet and finish in the oven at 350°F.
7. Transfer chicken thighs to a plate lined with paper towels.
8. Serve with ranch or dipping sauce or as is. Refrigerate or freeze in airtight containers or heavy-duty freezer bag for up to 4 months.

Bacon, Avocado, and Chicken Sandwich

Ingredients (1 serving):
- 1 serving cloud bread (see Easy Cloud Bread)
- 1 tablespoon mayonnaise
- 1 teaspoon sriracha
- 2 slices bacon
- 3 ounces chicken breast or other meat pieces
- 2 slices pepper jack cheese
- 2 whole grape tomatoes
- 1/2 avocado

Instructions:
1. Prepare cloud bread (see Easy Cloud Bread) or use leftovers. If chicken is not cooked, season with salt and pepper to taste and cook in water or in a pan with some oil until cooked through.
2. Slice cloud bread in half and spread mayonnaise and sriracha on both halves on the cut side. Cut grape tomatoes in half and mash avocado with a fork.
3. Place chicken on top of one half over mayonnaise, then top with cheese slices, bacon, and halved grape tomatoes.
4. Finish with spreading the mashed avocado on top and seasoning with salt if desired.
5. Cover the sandwich with the other halve of the cloud bread (mayo side down).
6. Enjoy!

Beef and Chicken Meatballs

Ingredients (5 servings):
- 1 ½ pounds lean grass fed ground beef
- ½ pound pastured chicken livers
- 1/2 large shallot
- 2 medium carrots
- 1 1/2 garlic cloves
- 1 tablespoon grass fed butter
- ½ teaspoon dried oregano
- 1 tablespoon coconut aminos, divided
- ½ tablespoon apple cider vinegar
- 1 ½ teaspoons salt, divided
- 1 teaspoon black pepper
- ½ tablespoon dried thyme (dried)
- ½ tablespoon garlic powder
- Olive oil

Instructions:
1. Finely mince shallots, carrots and garlic.
2. Heat a large cast iron skillet over medium heat until hot, then add butter, shallots, carrots and garlic and sauté, stirring frequently, for about 8 minutes or until fragrant and tender.
3. Add chicken livers 1/2 teaspoon salt and oregano and cook, stirring frequently, until livers are browned on all sides. Stir in ½ tablespoon coconut aminos and ½ tablespoon apple cider vinegar and cook until livers are cooked through.
4. Remove skillet from heat and when livers have cooled a little, transfer into a food processor. Pulse until looks like ground beef and let cool in a large bowl to a room temperature.
5. Preheat the oven to 425°F. Grease a baking sheet with olive oil.
6. Add ground beef to the liver along with remaining salt, thyme and garlic powder and stir until well incorporated. Form 1 1/2-inch balls, about 15 and coat them with oiled hands in little olive oil.
7. Place meatballs on the sheet and drizzle with reserved coconut aminos. Bake for 5 minutes at 425°F, then for 20 minutes at 350°F.
8. Serve right away with ranch, guacamole or drizzled with lemon tahini sauce, if desired. Refrigerate or freeze leftovers.

Easy Side Dishes and Snacks. Creamy Garlic Mashed Cauliflower

Ingredients (1 serving):

- 5 ounces cauliflower florets
- 1 teaspoon butter
- 1 tablespoon sour cream
- Salt to taste
- 2 tablespoons parmesan cheese
- 1/2 bulb garlic (2 to 3 cloves or to taste)
- 1/2 teaspoon olive oil

Instructions:

1. Preheat the oven to 300°F.
2. Divide garlic bulb in half and cut off the top. Drizzle with olive oil and roast in the oven for 25 minutes. When roasted, remove and carefully squeeze out garlic cloves.
3. Bring a pot of water to boil. Meanwhile, break cauliflower into florets and then add to the water. Boil for 5 minutes or until tender.
4. Drain cauliflower and place in a bowl. Add butter, sour cream, salt, and parmesan cheese and blend until pureed and smooth.
5. Serve and refrigerate leftovers for 4 to 5 days.

Arugula, Asparagus and Avocado Salad

Ingredients (1 serving):

- 10-12 stalks asparagus
- ½ tablespoon olive oil
- Salt and pepper, to taste
- 1 cup arugula
- 1/2 cup microgreens
- 1/2 avocado
- 1 egg
- 2 tablespoons sunflower seeds

Lemon vinaigrette:

- 1 tablespoon olive oil
- 1 ½ teaspoons lemon juice
- ½ teaspoon shallot, finely diced
- 1/8 teaspoon Dijon mustard
- Salt and pepper, to taste

Instructions:

1. Wash and trim the ends of asparagus, then cut into 1 to 1 ½ inch pieces.
2. Add olive oil to a small pan and heat over medium high heat. Add asparagus and season with salt and pepper to taste. Cook for 2 to 4 minutes, depending on the thickness of the stalks. Remove from heat and set aside.
3. Add water to a small pot and bring to boil over high heat. Lower the heat to simmering and carefully lower an egg with a spoon into the pot. Cook for 6 ½ minutes for soft-boiled eggs or 7 to 7 ½ minutes for hard-boiled eggs. Turn up the heat until its boiling again.
4. Meanwhile, add ice and water to a bowl and when egg is ready cool in the iced water. Peel, once cooled, and cut in half.
5. In a small bowl, whisk together olive oil, lemon juice, finely diced shallot, Dijon mustard and salt and pepper.
6. Add arugula and microgreens to a salad bowl and top with asparagus and sunflower seeds. Add avocado and egg halves.
7. Serve drizzled with lemon vinaigrette.

Easy Everything Bagels

Ingredients (2 servings):

- 2 cups almond flour
- 1 tablespoon baking powder
- 1 teaspoon garlic powder
- 1 teaspoon onion powder
- 1 teaspoon dried Italian seasoning
- 3 large eggs, divided
- 3 cups shredded low moisture mozzarella cheese
- 5 tablespoons cream cheese
- 3 tablespoons Everything Bagel Seasoning

For Everything Bagel Seasoning (1 cup):

- 1/4 cup toasted sesame seeds
- 3 tablespoons, plus 1 teaspoon poppy seeds
- 3 tablespoons, plus 1 teaspoon dried minced onions
- 3 tablespoons, plus 1 teaspoon dried garlic flakes
- 2 tablespoons coarse sea salt

Instructions:

1. Place toasted sesame seeds, poppy seeds, dried minced onions, dried garlic flakes into an airtight container or spice jar and shake to mix. Shake again before using.
2. Preheat oven to 425°F. Line a rimmed baking sheet with parchment paper.
3. Add almond flour, baking powder, garlic powder, onion powder, and dried Italian seasoning to a bowl and stir well together or sift together through flour sifter.
4. Add 1 egg to a small bowl and whisk with a fork to break up the egg white and yolk. Set aside.
5. Place mozzarella cheese and cream cheese into a microwave safe bowl and microwave for 1 ½ minutes. Stir and microwave for another minute. Stir again to mix cheeses together.
6. Add the other 2 eggs and cheeses and mix to form a dough. If it is too stringy, microwave for 30 seconds to soften the cheeses.
7. Roll 6 balls from the dough, then press in the center to form a ring. Stretch the ring to create a small hall in the center.
8. Brush the top of all bagels with the beaten egg and sprinkle with the seasoning. Bake for 12 to 14 minutes or until golden brown.
9. Serve.

Herb Salmon Salad

Ingredients (2 servings):

- 1 8-ounce salmon fillet
- Pinch of Himalayan rock salt
- Dash of freshly ground pepper
- 1/4 English cucumber, cut in half lengthwise then sliced
- 1/2 tomato, diced
- 2 sticks celery, diced
- 1 green onion, finely chopped

Dressing:

- 1 tablespoon fresh lemon juice
- 1 tablespoon extra virgin olive oil
- 1 tablespoon gluten-free Dijon mustard
- 1 tablespoon water
- 1 clove garlic
- 1 sprig fresh rosemary leaves
- 2 bunches fresh thyme leaves
- Pinch sea salt
- Freshly ground pepper
- 1/2 teaspoon black mustard seeds
- 2 tablespoons flat leaf parsley, roughly chopped

Instructions:

1. Preheat an oven broiler. Line a baking sheet with aluminum foil.
2. Set salmon fillet onto a baking sheet and season with salt and pepper. Place in the oven about 4 to 5 inches away from broiler and cook for about 10 minutes per every inch of thickness and about 5 to 8 minutes for thinner fillet, until the top is golden brown. Remove salmon and set aside to cool.
3. Meanwhile, cut cucumber in half lengthwise and slice, dice tomato and celery stick and finely chop green onion. Break salmon into pieces and add to a large bowl along with vegetables.
4. Add lemon juice, olive oil, Dijon mustard, water, garlic, rosemary leave, thyme, sea salt, and pepper to a food processor and pulse until smooth.
5. Add dressing to the salad and sprinkle with fresh chopped parsley and black mustard seeds.
6. Serve.

No-Bake Protein Bars

Ingredients (6 servings):
- 1/2 cup flax seed meal (grind whole flax in a coffee grinder)
- 2 tablespoons coconut flour
- 2 tablespoons sesame seeds
- 10 tablespoons protein powder
- 3 tablespoons carob powder
- 1/8 teaspoon stevia powder (or to taste)
- 1/3 cup almond butter, room temperature
- 2 tablespoons coconut oil, room temperature.
- 1 teaspoon vanilla extract
- 1/2 cup water (more or less, as necessary)

Instructions:
1. Place flax seed meal, coconut flour, sesame seeds, protein powder, carob powder, and stevia powder into a mixing bowl and stir to combine.
2. Mix together almond butter and coconut oil in a small bowl and add to the flour mixture. Stir with clean hands, if preferred, until well incorporated.
3. Add vanilla extract and a little water and mix again. Add enough water until no longer crumbly and dry.
4. Grease about a 9 by 9-inch pan and press the dough well into the pan, making sure the top is even. Refrigerate for several hours and then cut into six bars.
5. Enjoy!Wrap each one individually for a quick snackor store with wax paper in-between.

Satisfying Cheddar Chips

Ingredients (1 serving):
- 4 tablespoons Cheddar cheese, shredded
- Seasoning of choice (optional, not included in macros)

Instructions:
1. Preheat oven to 375°F. Line a cookie sheet with parchment paper
2. Place dollops of shredded Cheddar cheese (1 tablespoon each) about 2 inches apart onto the prepared cookie sheet. Sprinkle with seasoning of choice, if desired.
3. Place into the oven and bake for 10 to 15 minutes, until the edges are golden brown.
4. Remove from the oven and let cool for 10 to 15 minutes before loosening from the sheet with the help of a knife, if necessary.
5. Enjoy!

Avocado Chia Salad

Ingredients (1 serving):

- 1 ripe avocado, cut into cubes
- 1 tablespoon nutritional yeast
- ½ tablespoon chia seeds
- 1 tablespoon hemp or sunflower seeds
- 1 tablespoon apple cider vinegar
- 2 tablespoons extra virgin olive oil
- ½ tablespoon fresh lime juice
- Pink Himalayan salt to taste
- Pepper to taste

Instructions:

1. Cut avocado in half and remove the seed. Cut each half into cubes by cutting lengthwise and then across. Scoop out the cubed flesh with a spoon into a bowl.
2. Add nutritional yeast, chia seeds, and hemp or sunflower seeds. Drizzle with apple cider vinegar, extra virgin olive oil and fresh lime juice.
3. Season with salt and pepper and mix together.
4. Serve right away or refrigerate for up to 24 hours. Discard if avocado gets brown and moldy.

Cauliflower Fried Rice with Bacon

Ingredients (2 servings):
- 3 slices bacon, chopped
- 1/2 small onion, finely minced
- ½ medium head cauliflower, grated
- 1/2 tablespoon water
- 1/2 cup frozen mixed vegetables
- 1/2 tablespoon coconut aminosor fish sauce
- Seasoning of choice, to taste

Instructions:
1. Chop bacon, finely mince onion and grate cauliflower (or process in a food processor until resembles rice).
2. Heat a wok or large sauté pan over medium heat and add bacon. Cook until almost crispy.
3. Add onion and stir fry until the onion is translucent. Turn up the heat to high and add cauliflower. Stir fry for another minute.
4. Stir in water and mixed vegetables and cook, covered, for about 3 minutes or until vegetables are tender.
5. Add seasoning to taste and toss to mix together.
6. Serve.

Lemon Tuna Salad

- 1/3 cucumber, diced small
- 1/2 small avocado, diced small
- 1 teaspoon lemon juice
- 1 can (4-6 ounces) tuna
- 1 tablespoon mayonnaise or olive oil
- 1 tablespoon mustard
- Salt to taste
- Salad greens (optional)
- Black pepper to taste

Instructions:

1. Finely dice cucumber and avocado. Add lemon juice and stir to coat.
2. Flake tuna and stir in mayonnaise and mustard.
3. Add tuna mixture to the cucumber and avocado. Season salad with salt to taste.
4. Place salad greens on a serving plate, if using, and sprinkle with some olive oil and lemon juice, if desired.
5. Top greens with tuna salad and sprinkle with black pepper.
6. Serve.

Lebanese Tabbouleh Salad

Ingredients (1 serving):

- 1 tablespoon chia seeds
- 1 cups finely chopped parsley, stalks discarded
- 1large tomato, finely chopped
- 1 spring onion, finely chopped
- 2 mint leaves, finely chopped
- 3 tablespoons olive oil
- 1 tablespoon freshly squeezed lemon juice
- 1 teaspoon roasted cumin powder

Instructions:

1. Place chia seeds into a small bowl and soak in water for 10 minutes.
2. Meanwhile, whisk together lemon juice, olive oil and roasted cumin powder in a large bowl.
3. Finely chop tomato, spring onionand mint leaves. Add tomato, spring onion and mint leaves to the dressing and stir to combine.
4. Finely chop parsley leaves and strain water from the chia seeds.
5. Add parsley and chia seeds to the rest of the salad and toss to coat in dressing.
6. Serve sprinkled with unsoaked chia seeds and sprinkled with a pinch of salt.

Turkey Roll Ups

Ingredients (1 serving):

- 2 slices deli turkey breast
- 1/2 tablespoon garlic flavored hummus
- 1 tablespoon crumbled feta cheese
- 1 slice tomato, chopped up
- 3 pitted Greek olives, chopped
- 1 - 2 baby spinach leaves, torn into smaller pieces

Instructions:

1. Chop tomato slice and Greek olives. Tear spinach leaves into small pieces.
2. Place turkey slices on top of each other and top with hummus. Spread it over the turkey slices.
3. Add crumbled feta cheese, tomato, olives and spinach leaves on top and roll up. Cut roll in half.
4. Serve. If desired, make 1 to 2 days ahead and refrigerate in airtight container.

Quail Egg Salad

Ingredients (1 serving):

- 5 quail eggs, boiled and peeled
- 4 grape tomatoes
- 1/3 head butter lettuce, chopped into large pieces
- 2 1/2 slices crispy bacon, crumbled
- Olive oil and balsamic vinegar to taste
- Salt to taste

Instructions:

1. Bring a pot of water to boil and carefully add quail eggs. Boil for 3 minutes for soft boiled eggs or 4 to 5 minutes for hard boiled eggs. Remove and cool under cold water.
2. Meanwhile, if necessary, cook bacon on a skillet until crispy, let cool and crumble. Chop butter lettuce into large pieces.
3. Peel quail eggs and rinse off any remaining shell particles. Cut in half, if desired.
4. Add tomatoes, lettuce, and bacon to a salad bowl. Sprinkle with olive oil, balsamic vinegar and salt and toss together.
5. Place quail eggs on top or toss carefully, if desired.
6. Serve.

Cauliflower "Mac" and Cheese Casserole

Ingredients (4 servings):

- Kosher salt, as needed, plus 1/2 teaspoon
- 1 large head cauliflower, cut into small florets
- Vegetable oil spray
- 1 cup heavy cream
- 2 ounces cream cheese, cut into small pieces
- 1 1/2 teaspoons Dijon mustard
- 1 1/2 cups shredded sharp Cheddar, plus 1/2 cup for topping the casserole
- 1/4 teaspoon freshly ground black pepper
- 1/8 teaspoon garlic powder

Instructions:

1. Preheat oven to 375°F. Grease 4 mini aluminum pans with vegetable oil spray.
2. Add water and some salt to a large pot and bring to boil. Meanwhile, cut cauliflower into small florets and add to the boiling water. Cook for about 5 minutes until tender, but still crispy.
3. Drain cauliflower and set on paper towels to remove excess moisture. Divide among 4 pans and set aside.
4. Cut cream cheese into small pieces. Add heavy cream to a small saucepan and bring to simmer. Stir in cream cheese and mustard until smooth.
5. Add 1 ½ cups Cheddar cheese, salt, pepper and garlic powder and stir for 1 to 2 minutes, until the cheese melts. Pour the mixture over cauliflower, evenly dividing it.
6. Sprinkle with reserved Cheddar cheese and bake for about 15 minutes, until top is browned and cheese is bubbly. Alternatively, freeze each portion, covered tightly with aluminum foil, for up to 2 months. Then bake, frozen and covered and uncover at the end to brown the top.
7. Serve right away and refrigerate leftovers in airtight containers for up to 4 days.

Stacked Caprese Salad

Ingredients:

- 1/2 large tomato, cut into ½ inch slices
- 2 ounces fresh mozzarella cheese, cut into ½ inch slices
- ½ tablespoon olive oil
- ½ tablespoon balsamic reduction
- 2 basil leaves
- Pinch salt
- Pinch black pepper

Instructions:

1. Cut tomato and fresh mozzarella cheese into ½ inch slices. Alternatively, cut tomato and fresh mozzarella cheese into cubes.
2. Place tomato and mozzarella cheese slices, alternating the two, or cut into cubes just toss both in a salad bowl.
3. Season tomato and mozzarella cheese with salt and pepper and drizzle with olive oil and balsamic reduction to your taste.
4. Garnish salad with basil leaves.
5. Serve.

Bacon Spinach Salad

Ingredients (1 serving):

For the salad:

- ½ cup raw, washed spinach
- 1 ounce white mushrooms, sliced
- 2 ounces bacon, plus drippings
- ½ tablespoon red onion, finely diced
- 1 hard-boiled egg
- 1 ½ teaspoons olive oil
- ½ tablespoon slivered almonds

For the dressing:

- ½ -1 tablespoon bacon grease
- 1 teaspoon Dijon mustard
- 1 teaspoon red wine vinegar
- Salt and pepper
- ½ teaspoon chopped shallots
- Pinch sweetener (optional)

Instructions:

1. Preheat the oven to 375°F. Line a baking sheet with parchment paper.
2. Lay bacon on the baking sheet and cook in the oven for 15 to 18 minutes, until desired crispiness. Drain bacon grease into a small bowl and set aside.
3. Peel and slice hard boiled eggs (boil for 10 minutes) into thin slices. Finely dice shallot and red onion and slice mushrooms.
4. Add olive oil to a small saucepan and heat over medium heat. Add half of the shallots and cook for 1 minutes or until fragrant. Stir in mushrooms and cook until browned on both sides, 3 to 5 minutes.
5. Add spinach to a large bowl and top with crumbled bacon, mushrooms, red onion, egg and almonds.
6. In a separate bowl stir together vinegar and mustard. Add the other half of the cooked shallots and sweetener, if desired, and whisk together. Continue whisking and drizzle in warm bacon grease. Season with salt and pepper to taste. Add dressing to the salad.
7. Serve.

Mixed Green Spring Salad

Ingredients (1 serving):
- 2 ounces mixed greens
- 3 tablespoons roasted pine nuts
- 2 tablespoons raspberry vinaigrette
- 2 tablespoons shaved Parmesan
- 4 tablespoons shredded mozzarella cheese
- 2 slices bacon
- Salt and pepper to taste

Instructions:
1. Heat a skillet and cook bacon slices until very crispy.
2. Place mixed greens in a container with lid.
3. Add roasted pine nuts, vinaigrette, parmesan, mozzarella cheese, and crumbled bacon to the greens.
4. Cover with a lid and shake to coat and mix together. Transfer to a plate.
5. Serve.

Easy Cloud Bread

Ingredients (3 servings):

- 1 eggs room temperature
- 1 tablespoon cream cheese, softened
- Pinch cream of tartar
- Pinch salt

Instructions:

1. Preheat the oven to 300°F. Line a baking sheet parchment paper.
2. Separate egg and place white and yolk in different bowls.
3. Add cream cheese to the egg yolk and mix well with a hand mixer.
4. Add cream of tartar and salt to the egg white and beat with a hand mixer on high speed until stiff peaks form.
5. Carefully fold the yolk mixture into the egg white until well incorporated.
6. Spoon the mixture onto a baking sheet about ½ to ¾ inches tall and about 5 inches apart.
7. Bake for ½ hour or until tops are lightly golden. Remove from the oven and allow to cool.
8. Serve as desired.

Chicken and Celery Salad

Ingredients (1 serving):

- ¼ pound chicken breast
- 1/2 rib celery, diced
- 4 teaspoons mayonnaise
- 1/3 teaspoon brown mustard
- Pinch pink Himalayan salt
- 1/3 tablespoon fresh dill, chopped
- 1/3 ounce chopped pecans

Instructions:

1. Preheat the oven to 450°F. Line a baking sheet with parchment paper.
2. Place chicken breast onto a baking sheet and bake for about 15 minutes or until cooked through. Remove chicken and let cool completely.
3. Meanwhile, dice celery. Cut chicken into bite-size pieces.
4. Add chicken, celery, mayo, brown mustard, and salt to a large bowl and toss to mix everything and coat chicken in dressing.
5. Cover salad with a lid or plastic wrap and let chill in refrigerator for 1 to 2 hours. Meanwhile, chop fresh dill and pecans and set aside.
6. Right before serving, add fresh dill and pecans and toss to combine.
7. Serve.

Quick Zucchini Noodles

Ingredients (1 serving):

- 2 medium zucchini, spiralized
- ½ tablespoon oil or butter
- Salt and pepper to taste
- 1/3 teaspoon Parmesan cheese

Instructions:

1. Spiralize zucchini using a mandoline or julienne peeler. Place zucchini noodles between paper towels and squeeze as much liquid as you can.
2. Place noodles into a colander and season with salt. Set aside for 15 minutes for extra liquid to drain.
3. Add oil to a skillet and heat over high heat. Use paper towels to remove any excess moisture from zucchini noodles and add them to the skillet. Toss to coat in oil or butter and fry, stirring, for 1 to 2 minutes.
4. Serve with favorite sauce or ragout.

Perfect Caesar Salad

Ingredients (1 serving):

- 5⅓ ounces chicken breasts
- ½ tablespoon olive oil
- Salt and pepper
- 2⅔ ounces bacon
- ¼ Romaine lettuce
- 1 ounce freshly grated parmesan cheese

For dressing:

- 4 tablespoons mayonnaise
- ½ tablespoon Dijon mustard
- ¼ lemon, zest and juice
- 1 tablespoon grated parmesan cheese
- 1 tablespoon finely chopped filets of anchovies
- Salt and pepper

Instructions:

1. Whisk together mayonnaise, Dijon mustard, lemon zest and juice, parmesan cheese, anchovies and salt and pepper (can use an immersion blender). Place in refrigerator until ready to use.
2. Preheat the oven to 400°F. Grease a baking sheet.
3. Place chicken breast onto a baking sheet and sprinkle with salt and pepper and drizzle with olive oil or melted butter. Bake for 20 minutes or until cooked through or cook on the stovetop, if preferred.
4. Meanwhile, add bacon to a skillet and fry until crisp. Set aside. Shred lettuce and add to a serving plate.
5. Remove chicken and when cooled a little slice and place on top of lettuce. Top with crumbled bacon and dressing.
6. Serve sprinkled with parmesan cheese.

Mouthwatering Desserts. Chocolate Fudge Protein Bars

Ingredients (8 servings):

- 2 ounces raw unsalted sunflower seeds
- 2 ounces sunbutter or tahini
- 1 scoop chocolate protein powder
- 1 1/2 ounces unsweetened cocoa powder
- 1 1/2 ouncespowdered sugar free sweetener
- 1/4 teaspoon salt
- 4 tablespoons softened coconut oil

Optional coating:

- 1/4 cup sugar free chocolate chips
- 1/2 tablespoon butter

Instructions:

1. Add sunflower seeds, sunbutter or tahini, chocolate protein powder, cocoa powder, sweetener, salt and softened coconut oil to a food processor.
2. Process, scraping up the sides couple times, until the mixture is smooth. Taste and add sweetener if desired.
3. Line a loaf pan with parchment paper and add batter to the pan. Even out the top and place in refrigerator for ½ hour.
4. Remove the pan and cut into 8 bars. If making a coating, then freeze bars for ½ hour.
5. To make the coating, place butter and melt chocolate chips into a microwave safe bowl and melt in microwave for 1 minute. Alternatively, melt on the stovetop. Stir until no lumps remain and the mixture is smooth.
6. Line a baking sheet with parchment paper. Dip the bottom half of the bars into the chocolate mixture and set on a baking sheet. If desired, drizzle leftover chocolate on top.
7. Enjoy! Store in airtight container in refrigerator.

Easy Banana Bread

Ingredients (7 slices):
- 3 1/2 eggs
- 1 cup almond flour
- 1/4 cup butter or 1/8 cup olive oil
- 1 tablespoon olive oil
- 1/8 cup sunflower seeds
- 1 tablespoon chia seeds
- 1/2 teaspoon baking powder
- 1/4 teaspoon xanthium gum
- Pinch salt
- 2 drops banana extract
- 1/8 cup erythritol
- 1 tablespoon sesame seeds (topping)

Instructions:
1. Preheat the oven to 355°F. Line a loaf pan with parchment paper.
2. To divide egg in half, whisk it and take 2 tablespoons for the recipe. Add eggs to a mixing bowl and beat on high speed for 1 to 2 minutes.
3. Continue beating and add olive oil and butter.
4. Add sunflower seeds, chia seeds, baking powder, xanthium gum, salt, banana extract and erythritol to the egg and oil mixture and beat to combine.
5. Transfer the batter into the pan and sprinkle the sesame seeds on top.
6. Bake for 45 minutes or until a toothpick inserted in the center comes out clean. Remove the banana bread and let cool completely before slicing (freeze the loaf partially for easier slicing).
7. Serve and freeze leftovers, with each piece wrapped in plastic wrap and place everything in one freezer storage bag. Freeze for up to 4 months and thaw in refrigerator or at room temperature.

Peanut Butter Protein Cookies

Ingredients (1 serving):

- 2 heaping tablespoons peanut butter
- 1/4 cup whey protein powder
- 1/4 cup coconut milk (or almond milk)
- 1/4 cup ground almonds
- 1/4 cup pea protein powder

Instructions:

1. Preheat the oven to 340°F.
2. Add peanut butter, whey protein powder, coconut or almond milk, ground almonds and pea protein powder to a mixing bowl. Stir until well combined and looks like dough.
3. Form six balls from the mixture and place onto a cookie tray (grease, if necessary). Flatten with your fingers or crosswise with a fork to make a pattern.
4. Place cookies into the oven and bake for 5 to 10 minutes, until feel cooked when pressed. Remove cookies from the oven and let cool completely.
5. Enjoy!

Egg Cream Smoothie

Ingredients (1 serving):

- 2 raw eggs
- 2 tablespoons cream cheese
- ¼ cup heavy cream
- 1 tablespoon sugar-free vanilla syrup
- 3 ice cubes

Instructions:

1. Add eggs, cream cheese, heavy cream, vanilla syrup and ice cubes to a high-power blender.
2. Blend until well combined and almost smooth consistency.
3. Pour smoothie into a serving glass.
4. Enjoy!

Avocado, Chia Seeds and Cacao Smoothie

Ingredients (1 serving):

- ½ -3/4 cup full-fat coconut milk
- 1/2 frozen avocado
- 1/2 tablespoon nut butter of choice
- 1/2 tablespoon chia seeds, soaked
- 1 1/2 scoops chocolate protein powder
- 1/2 tablespoon coconut oil
- Ice (optional)
- Cacao nibs and cinnamon, for topping
- ¼ cup water, if needed

Instructions:

1. Soak chia seeds in 3 tablespoons of water for 10 minutes.
2. Place coconut milk, avocado, nut butter of choice, chia seeds, chocolate protein powder, coconut oil, and ice (if desired) into a high-powered blender. If needed, add some water.
3. Blend all the ingredients until well combined.
4. Transfer into a serving glass and sprinkle with cacao nibs and cinnamon.
5. Enjoy!

Avocado Chocolate Pudding

Ingredients (1 serving):

- 1/2 medium ripe avocado
- 1/8 cup cocoa powder
- 5 drops stevia
- 1/4 teaspoon vanilla extract
- Mint leaves for garnishing

Instructions:

1. Cut avocado in half and remove the seed. Scrape out the flesh into a medium bowl.
2. Using a fork slightly mash the avocado.
3. Add cocoa powder, stevia and vanilla extract. Use fork to incorporate everything together and at the same time mash avocado until it looks like pudding. If desired, use an electric mixer to quicken the process.
4. Serve garnished with mint leaves.

Moist and Soft Vanilla Cake

Ingredients (3 servings):
Cake:

- 1 ounceerythritol
- 1 ouncebutter (softened)
- 1 large egg
- 1 tablespoonunsweetened almond milk
- 1/3 teaspoonvanilla extract
- 6 tablespoonsalmond flour
- 1 tablespooncoconut flour
- 2/3 teaspoon baking powder

Cream cheese frosting:

- 4 ounces cream cheese (softened)
- 2/3 tablespoon butter (softened)
- 1 ½ tablespoons powdered erythritol
- 1/3 teaspoon vanilla extract

Instructions:
1. Preheat the oven to 350°F. Line a bottom of a small pan with parchment paper and grease the sides.
2. Place butter and erythritol into a large bowl and beat with a mixer until fluffy. Add egg, beat and then add almond milk and vanilla extract.
3. Add almond flour, coconut flour and baking powder and beat until incorporated.
4. Add 1/3 or ½ of the dough (depending on the desired number and thickness of cake layers) to the pan and smooth the top with a spatula.
5. Bake cake layer for 15 to 20 minutes, or until the top is lightly golden and springy when touched. Repeat with remaining batter. Allow layers to cool separately to room temperature.
6. While cake layers are baking and cooling, add cream cheese, butter, powdered erythritol and vanilla extract to a mixing bowl and beat together until smooth.
7. Frost the cake layers and the top and sides at the end with cream cheese frosting. If desired, add chopped nuts to the top or sides.
8. Serve. Refrigerate for 5 to 6 days.

Chocolate Peanut Butter Cake

Ingredients (1 serving):
- 1 tablespoon peanut butter
- 1 large egg
- 2 tablespoons butter
- 3 tablespoons heavy whipping cream
- 1 tablespoon powdered stevia
- 1/2 teaspoon baking powder
- 1 1/2 tablespoons unsweetened cocoa powder
- 1/2 teaspoon vanilla extract
- Pinch of salt

Instructions:
1. Add butter to a mug or a ramekin and melt in microwave on high in 30 seconds intervals, until almost fully melted.
2. Add stevia, cocoa powder, baking powder and salt to the butter and stir to combine.
3. Crack egg into a mixer bowl. Using a hand beater or electric mixer beat together on medium high speed with 1 tablespoon heavy whipping cream until small bubbles appear.
4. Add egg and cream mixture to the butter along with vanilla extract and whisk it together, getting more air into the batter.
5. Add a peanut butter into the center of the batter, submerging it under the mixture slightly so it's surrounded with batter on all sides.
6. Place into a microwave and cook for 1 minutes. Carefully flip the cake onto a serving plate (use a butter knife to separate it from the edges, if necessary).
7. Enjoy with remaining whipping cream!

Conclusion

We hope that this book proved that aside from having many health benefits, keto diet can be very delicious, and you will never experience a feeling of hunger on it. With the help of such nutritional plan, the thought of recharging with a doughnut or a chocolate bar is unlikely to come to anyone's head. On the ketogenic diet, as you likely realized, overall well-being and emotional state improve, energy levels increase, the brain starts to work at the speed of light and the concentration of attention increases. To keep you more motivated, we would also like to point out the following:

➢ Restriction of carbohydrates is the most effective way to reduce blood sugar.
➢ Restriction of carbohydrates is beneficial for health even without weight loss.
➢ The volume all fats and saturated fats consumed does not correlate with the risks of cardiovascular diseases.
➢ Limiting the intake of carbohydrates is the most effective way (with the exception of fasting) of lowering the level of triglycerides and increasing the level of high-density lipoproteins (the so-called "good cholesterol" - HDL).

Finally, we hope that no matter why your decided to follow a keto diet, you are able to achieve your goals and enjoy your time with this meal plan. We are sure that you will be able to effortlessly cook and then savor every dish with the help of the easy to follow recipes we included in this book. Happy cooking and stay healthy!